Unmasking the Silent Killer

Heart Disease

Logan Smith

Copyright © (Logan Smith) 2023. All rights reserved

The reproduction or duplication of this document is prohibited without the publisher's consent. Any electronic storage, transfer, or inclusion in a database is also prohibited. The document cannot be copied, scanned, faxed, or retained in part or in full without approval from the publisher or creator.

Table of Contents

Introduction

In the depths of our bodies, concealed beneath the veil of normalcy, a silent killer lies in wait. Its name is heart disease, a stealthy adversary that claims countless lives, often without warning. While it may remain unseen, its impact reverberates through individuals, families, and communities, leaving behind a trail of shattered dreams and unfulfilled potential.

Heart disease, encompassing a range of conditions that afflict the heart and blood vessels, is a formidable foe. From coronary artery disease to heart failure, arrhythmias to valvular abnormalities, its manifestations are diverse and its consequences dire. Yet, it has long been shrouded in secrecy, eluding detection until it strikes with devastating force.

But today, we embark on a journey to unmask this silent killer. We step into the light of awareness, armed with knowledge and determination. No longer will heart disease thrive in the shadows of ignorance and indifference. Together, we will unravel its mysteries, expose its insidious ways, and forge a path towards prevention, treatment, and a brighter future.

In this exploration, we will delve into the causes and risk factors that lay the groundwork for heart disease's infiltration. We will examine the signs and symptoms that offer subtle hints of its presence, as well as the diagnostic tests and procedures that enable its detection. We will explore the treatment options available to those affected, from lifestyle modifications to advanced interventions, and the innovative research shaping the future of cardiovascular care.

Moreover, we will emphasize the importance of preventing the shield that guards against heart disease's encroachment. By understanding the critical role of a healthy diet, regular exercise, and stress management, we can fortify ourselves against this stealthy adversary. We will unravel the interplay of genetics, lifestyle choices, and environmental factors, unveiling the complexities of heart disease's grip.

Through this journey, we will confront the emotional and psychological impact that heart disease imposes on individuals and their loved ones. We will uncover the support systems and resources available to navigate the challenges, while also acknowledging the importance of cardiac rehabilitation programs in fostering recovery and resilience.

Unmasking the silent killer is not a task for the faint-hearted. It requires a collective commitment to prioritize heart health, to seek knowledge, and to take action. Together, let us strip away the cloak of mystery, empowering ourselves and our communities to stand against heart disease. By raising awareness, advocating for change, and embracing heart-healthy habits, we can shift the narrative and reclaim our lives from the clutches of this silent killer.

Chapter 1

Overview

Heart disease, also known as cardiovascular disease, refers to a range of conditions that affect the heart and blood vessels. It is a broad term encompassing various disorders such as coronary artery disease, heart failure, arrhythmias, and valvular heart disease. These conditions can have a significant impact on an individual's health and quality of life, and they remain a leading cause of death worldwide.

Prevalence

Heart disease is a global health concern, affecting individuals of all ages and backgrounds. According to the World Health Organization (WHO), cardiovascular diseases account for approximately 17.9 million deaths each year, representing 31% of all global deaths. This staggering statistic highlights the urgent need for preventive measures and effective management of heart disease.

The prevalence of heart disease varies across different regions and populations. It is more common in developed countries due to factors such as sedentary lifestyles, unhealthy diets, and aging populations.

However, there is also an increasing prevalence in developing countries as they undergo socioeconomic transitions, leading to lifestyle changes and an increase in risk factors.

Impact

The impact of heart disease extends beyond mortality rates. It poses a substantial burden on healthcare systems, economies, and individuals' quality of life. Heart disease can lead to severe complications such as heart attacks, strokes, heart failure, and reduced physical activity.

Heart attacks, or myocardial infarctions, occur when there is a sudden blockage in the coronary arteries, cutting off the blood supply to the heart. This can result in permanent damage to the heart muscle and, in some cases, can be fatal. Strokes, on the other hand, occur when the blood supply to the brain is interrupted, leading to brain cell damage. Both heart attacks and strokes can cause long-term disabilities and significantly impact an individual's ability to perform daily activities.

Heart failure is a chronic condition in which the heart cannot pump enough blood to meet the body's needs. It can lead to symptoms such as fatigue, shortness of breath, and fluid retention, impairing an individual's ability to engage in physical activities and affecting their overall quality of life.

In addition to the physical and emotional impact on individuals, heart disease also places a substantial burden on healthcare systems. The cost of managing heart disease, including hospitalizations, medications, surgeries, and rehabilitation, is substantial. This burden is expected to increase as the global population ages and risk factors such as obesity and diabetes continue to rise.

Risk Factors

Several risk factors contribute to the development of heart disease, including:

Unhealthy Lifestyle

Poor diet, lack of physical activity, smoking, excessive alcohol consumption, and obesity increase the risk of heart disease. Diets high in saturated and trans fats, cholesterol, and sodium can contribute to the development of atherosclerosis, a condition characterized by the buildup of plaque in the arteries.

Age and Gender

The risk of heart disease increases with age. Men are generally at a higher risk than pre-menopausal women; however, after menopause, women's risk catches up to that of men. Estrogen provides some protection against heart disease in pre-menopausal women.

Family History

A family history of heart disease, especially if a close relative developed it at an early age, increases the risk. Genetic factors play a role in the development of heart disease, although lifestyle factors also contribute significantly.

High Blood Pressure

Hypertension is a significant risk factor for heart disease, as it strains the heart and damages blood vessels. Persistent high blood pressure can lead to the thickening and narrowing of arteries, increasing the risk of heart attacks and strokes.

High Cholesterol Levels

Elevated levels of cholesterol, particularly LDL (bad) cholesterol, can lead to the formation of plaques in the arteries, restricting blood flow to the heart. This condition, known as coronary artery disease, is a common form of heart disease.

Diabetes

Individuals with diabetes are at an increased risk of developing heart disease due to the impact of high blood sugar on blood vessels. Diabetes can also contribute to the development of other risk factors such as obesity and high blood pressure.

Stress and Mental Health

Chronic stress, depression, and anxiety have been associated with an increased risk of heart disease. These factors can contribute to unhealthy behaviors such as overeating, smoking, and physical inactivity.

Other Medical Conditions

Certain conditions like obesity, metabolic syndrome, sleep apnea, and chronic kidney disease can contribute to the development of heart disease. These conditions often coexist with other risk factors and can further increase the likelihood of cardiovascular complications.

Understanding these risk factors is crucial for prevention, early detection, and effective management of heart disease. Adopting a heart-healthy lifestyle, managing stress, regular exercise, maintaining a balanced diet, and regular check-ups can significantly reduce the risk of developing heart disease.

In summary, heart disease is a broad term encompassing various conditions affecting the heart and blood vessels. It is a global health concern with significant prevalence and impact on mortality, healthcare systems, and individuals' well-being. Awareness, prevention, and management strategies are essential to reduce the burden of heart disease and improve overall cardiovascular health. By addressing risk factors and promoting healthy lifestyles, individuals can take proactive steps toward preventing heart disease and maintaining a healthy heart.

Chapter 2

Anatomy and Function of the Heart

The heart is a vital organ located in the chest cavity, slightly to the left. It is a muscular pump responsible for circulating oxygenated blood to all parts of the body. The heart consists of four chambers: two upper chambers called atria (singular: atrium) and two lower chambers called ventricles. The chambers are separated by a muscular wall called the septum.

Functionally, the heart acts as a double pump. The right side of the heart receives deoxygenated blood from the body and pumps it to the lungs for oxygenation. The left side of the heart receives oxygenated blood from the lungs and pumps it to the rest of the body.

Structure of the Heart

Atria

The right atrium receives deoxygenated blood from the body through two large veins, the superior vena cava (which collects blood from the upper body) and the inferior vena cava (which collects blood from the lower body). The left atrium receives oxygenated blood from the lungs through four pulmonary veins.

Ventricles

The right ventricle receives deoxygenated blood from the right atrium and pumps it to the lungs through the pulmonary artery. The left ventricle receives oxygenated blood from the left atrium and pumps it to the rest of the body through the largest artery, the aorta.

Valves

The heart has four valves that ensure one-way blood flow. The tricuspid valve separates the right atrium and right ventricle, while the mitral (or bicuspid) valve separates the left atrium and left ventricle. The pulmonary valve is located between the right ventricle and the pulmonary artery, and the aortic valve is located between the left ventricle and the aorta.

Circulatory System

The heart is a part of the circulatory system, also known as the cardiovascular system, which comprises blood vessels and blood. The circulatory system delivers oxygen, nutrients, hormones, and other essential substances to cells and carries away waste products.

The circulatory system consists of two main types of blood vessels:

Arteries

Arteries carry oxygenated blood (except for the pulmonary artery) away from the heart to the body's tissues. The aorta is the largest artery and branches into smaller arteries that reach various parts of the body.

Veins

Veins carry deoxygenated blood (except for the pulmonary veins) from the body's tissues back to the heart. The superior and inferior vena cava are the largest veins that return blood to the right atrium. The pulmonary veins carry oxygenated blood from the lungs to the left atrium.

The heart's Role in Blood Supply

The heart plays a crucial role in the circulation of blood. Deoxygenated blood returns to the heart through the superior and inferior vena cava, entering the right atrium. From there, it flows through the tricuspid valve into the right ventricle. The right ventricle then contracts, pumping the deoxygenated blood through the pulmonary valve into the pulmonary artery. The pulmonary artery carries the blood to the lungs, where it picks up oxygen and releases carbon dioxide. Oxygenated blood returns to the heart through the pulmonary veins, entering the left atrium. It then passes through the mitral valve into the left ventricle. The left ventricle contracts, pumping the oxygenated blood through the aortic valve into the aorta. From the aorta, the blood is distributed to the entire body through arteries, eventually reaching capillaries where oxygen and nutrients are exchanged with tissues. Deoxygenated blood returns to the heart through veins, and the cycle continues.

In summary, the heart is a complex organ responsible for pumping blood and maintaining circulation throughout the body. Its structure, consisting of four chambers and valves, allows for efficient and coordinated pumping action. The circulatory system, including arteries, veins, and capillaries, supports the heart's role in delivering oxygenated blood to tissues and removing waste products. Together, the heart and circulatory system ensure the continuous supply of oxygen and nutrients, supporting overall bodily functions.

Chapter 3

Types of Heart Disease

Coronary Artery Disease (CAD)

Coronary artery disease is the most common type of heart disease. It occurs when the arteries that supply blood to the heart become narrowed or blocked due to the buildup of fatty deposits called plaques. This restricts blood flow to the heart and can lead to chest pain (angina), heart attacks, and other complications.

Heart Failure

Heart failure is a condition in which the heart is unable to pump enough blood to meet the body's needs. It can occur when the heart muscles become weakened or stiff, often as a result of other conditions such as CAD, high blood pressure, or heart valve problems. Symptoms of heart failure include fatigue, shortness of breath, fluid retention, and reduced exercise tolerance.

Arrhythmias

Arrhythmias refer to abnormal heart rhythms. They occur when the electrical impulses that regulate the heart's pumping action are disrupted. Arrhythmias can cause the heart to beat too fast (tachycardia), too slow (bradycardia), or irregularly. While some arrhythmias are harmless, others can be life-threatening and require medical intervention.

Valvular Heart Disease

Valvular heart disease involves abnormalities or damage to the heart valves, which control blood flow through the heart. Conditions such as valve stenosis (narrowing) or valve regurgitation (leakage) can impair the heart's ability to pump blood efficiently. Valvular heart disease can be congenital or acquired through conditions such as infections or aging.

Congenital Heart Disease

Congenital heart disease refers to structural abnormalities in the heart that are present at birth. These abnormalities can affect the heart's walls, valves, or blood vessels. Congenital heart defects vary in severity, with some requiring immediate medical intervention and others causing minimal symptoms or complications.

Cardiomyopathy

Cardiomyopathy is a group of diseases that affect the heart muscle. It can cause the heart to become enlarged, thickened, or rigid, leading to reduced pumping ability. Cardiomyopathy can be inherited or acquired through factors such as infections, alcohol abuse, or certain medications.

Heart Infections

Heart infections, such as endocarditis or myocarditis, occur when the heart tissue or valves become inflamed due to a bacterial, viral, or fungal infection. These infections can interfere with normal heart function and may require antibiotics or other treatments.

It's important to note that these are just some of the many types of heart diseases that exist. Each condition has its own causes, symptoms, and treatment approaches. Diagnosis and management of heart disease should be done by qualified healthcare professionals based on individual circumstances and medical history.

Chapter 4

Causes and Risk Factors of Heart Disease

Atherosclerosis

Atherosclerosis is a major cause of heart disease. It occurs when fatty deposits, cholesterol, and other substances build up in the arteries, forming plaques. These plaques can narrow or block the arteries, reducing blood flow to the heart and increasing the risk of heart attacks and other cardiovascular complications.

Hypertension (High Blood Pressure)

High blood pressure is a significant risk factor for heart disease. When blood pressure remains consistently high, it puts strain on the arteries and the heart itself, increasing the risk of coronary artery disease, heart failure, and other cardiovascular problems.

High Cholesterol

Elevated levels of cholesterol, particularly low-density lipoprotein (LDL) cholesterol (often referred to as "bad" cholesterol), can contribute to the development of atherosclerosis. When LDL cholesterol levels are high, it can lead to the formation of plaques in the arteries, narrowing them and impairing blood flow to the heart.

Diabetes

Diabetes, especially type 2 diabetes, is a risk factor for heart disease. High blood sugar levels can damage blood vessels and contribute to the development of atherosclerosis. Individuals with diabetes also tend to have other risk factors such as obesity and high blood pressure, further increasing their risk of heart disease.

Obesity

Obesity is associated with an increased risk of heart disease. Excess body weight, especially around the abdomen, can lead to conditions such as high blood pressure, high cholesterol, and diabetes, all of which contribute to heart disease development.

Smoking and Tobacco Use

Smoking and tobacco use are major risk factors for heart disease. The chemicals in tobacco smoke damage blood vessels, reduce oxygen levels, promote the formation of blood clots, and contribute to the development of atherosclerosis. Secondhand smoke exposure can also increase the risk of heart disease.

Family History

Having a family history of heart disease, especially if a close relative developed it at an early age, increases the risk. Genetic factors can play a role in the development of heart disease, but lifestyle factors and shared environments within families can also contribute to the increased risk.

Other factors that can contribute to heart disease risk include a sedentary lifestyle, poor diet (high in saturated and trans fats, cholesterol, and sodium), excessive alcohol consumption, chronic stress, and certain medical conditions such as chronic kidney disease and sleep apnea.

It's important to note that while these risk factors can increase the likelihood of developing heart disease, they do not guarantee that an individual will develop it. Many heart disease cases are preventable or manageable through lifestyle modifications, medication, and other interventions. Regular medical check-ups, early detection, and adopting a heart-healthy lifestyle are crucial for reducing the risk of heart disease and promoting cardiovascular health.

Chapter 5

Signs, Symptoms, and Diagnosis of Heart Disease

Common Symptoms of Heart Disease

Chest Pain or Discomfort

Chest pain or discomfort, often described as pressure, tightness, or squeezing, is a common symptom of heart disease. It may radiate to the arm, jaw, neck, or back. This symptom, known as angina, can occur during physical exertion or stress and usually subsides with rest.

Shortness of Breath

Difficulty breathing or shortness of breath can occur with heart disease, particularly during physical activity or when lying flat. This symptom may be accompanied by a feeling of fatigue or inability to catch one's breath.

Fatigue

Unexplained fatigue or a feeling of tiredness can be a symptom of heart disease. The heart's reduced ability to pump blood efficiently can lead to inadequate oxygen supply to the muscles, resulting in fatigue.

Palpitations

Palpitations refer to a sensation of irregular, rapid, or pounding heartbeats. It can feel like the heart is skipping beats or beating too hard. Palpitations may be accompanied by dizziness or lightheadedness.

Swelling

Fluid retention, resulting in swelling of the legs, ankles, feet, or abdomen, can occur in heart disease. This swelling, known as edema, is caused by the heart's inability to effectively pump blood and fluid buildup in the body.

Dizziness or Fainting

Feeling lightheaded, dizzy, or experiencing fainting spells can be related to heart disease. These symptoms occur when there is inadequate blood flow to the brain due to a compromised heart function.

Diagnostic Tests and Procedures

Electrocardiogram (ECG/EKG)

An electrocardiogram is a non-invasive test that records the electrical activity of the heart. It can detect abnormal heart rhythms, signs of a previous heart attack, and other heart abnormalities.

Echocardiogram

An echocardiogram uses sound waves (ultrasound) to create images of the heart's structure and function. It provides detailed information about the heart's chambers, valves, and pumping ability.

Stress Test

A stress test, also known as an exercise stress test or treadmill test, evaluates the heart's response to physical exertion. It involves monitoring the heart's electrical activity while the person exercises on a treadmill or stationary bike.

Coronary Angiography

Coronary angiography is an invasive procedure that uses contrast dye and X-rays to visualize the coronary arteries. It helps identify blockages or narrowing in the arteries and determines the need for further intervention, such as angioplasty or stenting.

Blood Tests

Blood tests can assess various factors related to heart health, including cholesterol levels, blood sugar levels (for diabetes screening), and markers of inflammation or damage to the heart muscles.

Other diagnostic tests and procedures that may be used to evaluate heart disease include cardiac computed tomography (CT) scans, cardiac magnetic resonance imaging (MRI), Holter monitoring (continuous ECG recording over 24 hours), and nuclear stress tests.

It's important to consult with a healthcare professional for proper evaluation and diagnosis of heart disease. They will consider the individual's symptoms, medical history, risk factors, and the results of diagnostic tests to make an accurate diagnosis and develop an appropriate treatment plan.

Chapter 6

Treatment Options for Heart Disease

Lifestyle Modifications

Lifestyle changes play a key role in managing heart disease and reducing the risk of complications. These may include:

Adopting a heart-healthy diet

Emphasizing fruits, vegetables, whole grains, lean proteins, and limiting saturated fats, trans fats, sodium, and added sugars.

Regular physical activity

Engaging in regular exercise, as recommended by a healthcare professional, to improve cardiovascular fitness and overall health.

Smoking cessation

Quitting smoking and avoiding exposure to secondhand smoke.

Weight management

Achieving and maintaining a healthy weight through a combination of a balanced diet and regular physical activity.

Stress management

Implementing stress-reducing techniques such as relaxation exercises, meditation, or counseling.

Medications

Various medications may be prescribed to manage heart disease, depending on the specific condition and symptoms. These can include:

Statins

To lower cholesterol levels and reduce the risk of plaque buildup in the arteries.

Antiplatelet drugs

To prevent blood clots and reduce the risk of heart attacks or strokes.

Beta-blockers

To control blood pressure, reduce heart rate, and manage certain heart conditions.

Angiotensin-converting enzyme (ACE) inhibitors or angiotensin receptor blockers (ARBs)

To manage high blood pressure and heart failure.

Diuretics

To reduce fluid buildup and manage symptoms of heart failure.

Anticoagulants

To prevent blood clots in individuals with certain heart conditions.

Surgical Procedures

In some cases, surgical interventions may be necessary to treat heart disease. Common surgical procedures include:

Coronary artery bypass grafting (CABG)

A surgical procedure that bypasses blocked or narrowed coronary arteries by grafting healthy blood vessels from other parts of the body to restore blood flow to the heart.

Heart valve surgery

Repair or replacement of damaged or diseased heart valves to restore normal blood flow through the heart.

Cardiac transplant

In severe cases of heart failure, a heart transplant may be considered to replace a failing heart with a healthy donor heart.

Interventional Cardiology

Interventional cardiology procedures are minimally invasive techniques performed by specialized cardiologists. These procedures aim to diagnose and treat certain heart conditions without open surgery. Examples include:

Percutaneous coronary intervention (PCI)

A procedure to open blocked or narrowed coronary arteries using techniques such as balloon angioplasty and stenting.

Catheter-based valve procedures

Minimally invasive procedures to repair or replace heart valves using catheters, avoiding the need for open-heart surgery.

Cardiac Rehabilitation

Cardiac rehabilitation programs provide comprehensive support and guidance to individuals recovering from heart disease or cardiac procedures. These programs combine supervised exercise, education on heart-healthy lifestyle habits, and emotional support to improve overall cardiovascular health and quality of life.

The choice of treatment depends on the specific type and severity of heart disease, as well as individual factors such as overall health and medical history. Healthcare professionals, including cardiologists and cardiac surgeons, play a crucial role in determining the most appropriate treatment plan for each individual.

Chapter 7

Prevention and Risk Reduction for Heart Disease

Healthy Diet and Nutrition

Adopting a heart-healthy diet is crucial for preventing heart disease. This includes:

Consuming a variety of fruits, vegetables, whole grains, and lean proteins.

Limiting saturated fats, trans fats, cholesterol, sodium, and added sugars.

Choosing healthier cooking methods such as grilling, baking, or steaming instead of frying.

Monitoring portion sizes to maintain a healthy weight.

Regular Physical Activity

Engaging in regular physical activity helps maintain a healthy weight, lower blood pressure, improve cholesterol levels, and reduce the risk of heart disease. Aim for at least 150 minutes of moderate-intensity aerobic exercise or 75 minutes of vigorous-intensity aerobic exercise per week, along with strength training exercises twice a week.

Managing Blood Pressure and Cholesterol

High blood pressure and cholesterol are major risk factors for heart disease. To manage these:

Monitor blood pressure regularly and take prescribed medications as directed.

Follow a low-sodium diet, limit alcohol consumption, and manage stress to help control blood pressure.

Maintain healthy cholesterol levels by following a heart-healthy diet, taking prescribed cholesterol-lowering medications if needed, and getting regular cholesterol screenings.

Smoking Cessation

Quitting smoking and avoiding exposure to secondhand smoke is crucial for heart disease prevention. Seek support from healthcare professionals, join smoking cessation programs, and use medications or nicotine replacement therapies if necessary.

Diabetes Control

If you have diabetes, it's important to manage your blood sugar levels effectively to reduce the risk of heart disease. Follow your healthcare professional's recommendations for medication, monitoring, and lifestyle modifications to keep your diabetes under control.

Stress Management

Chronic stress can contribute to the development of heart disease. Implement stress-reducing techniques such as relaxation exercises, meditation, yoga, or engaging in activities that bring joy and relaxation. Seek support from friends, family, or professionals if needed.

Regular Health Check-ups

Schedule regular check-ups with your healthcare professional to assess your overall health and identify any risk factors or early signs of heart disease.

Follow their recommendations for screenings, vaccinations, and preventive measures.

It's important to remember that prevention and risk reduction strategies should be personalized based on individual needs and medical history. Consult with healthcare professionals, such as primary care physicians or cardiologists, for guidance and advice on implementing preventive measures tailored to your specific circumstances.

Chapter 8

Living with Heart Disease

Emotional and Psychological Impact

Heart disease can have a significant emotional and psychological impact on individuals. It can lead to feelings of anxiety, depression, fear, and frustration. It's important to recognize and address these emotions by seeking support from loved ones, joining support groups, or talking to a mental health professional. Open communication with healthcare providers can also help alleviate concerns and provide guidance.

Support Systems and Resources

Building a strong support system is essential when living with heart disease. Seek support from family, friends, and loved ones who can offer encouragement, understanding, and assistance. Additionally, there are numerous resources available, including patient advocacy groups, online forums, and educational materials, which provide valuable information and support for individuals with heart disease.

Cardiac Rehabilitation Programs

Cardiac rehabilitation programs are structured programs that offer support and guidance to individuals recovering from heart disease or cardiac procedures. These programs typically include exercise training, education on heart-healthy lifestyle habits, nutritional guidance, and emotional support. Participating in cardiac rehabilitation can improve physical fitness, reduce symptoms, and enhance overall well-being.

Lifestyle Changes for Better Heart Health

Adopting and maintaining a heart-healthy lifestyle is crucial when living with heart disease. This may include:

Following a nutritious, balanced diet low in saturated fats, trans fats, sodium, and added sugars.

Engaging in regular physical activity as recommended by healthcare professionals.

Taking prescribed medications consistently and following medication schedules.

Managing stress through relaxation techniques, mindfulness, and self-care practices.

Avoiding tobacco and limiting alcohol consumption.

Maintaining a healthy weight through portion control and regular exercise.

Monitoring and Follow-up Care

Regular monitoring and follow-up care are important aspects of managing heart disease. This includes:

Keeping appointments with healthcare professionals and following their recommendations.

Monitoring blood pressure, cholesterol levels, and other relevant parameters at home, as advised by healthcare providers.

Tracking and reporting any changes in symptoms or new symptoms to healthcare professionals.

Adhering to medication schedules and reporting any side effects to healthcare providers.

Attending regular check-ups, screenings, and tests as recommended.

By implementing these strategies and making necessary lifestyle changes, individuals living with heart disease can effectively manage their condition, reduce the risk of complications, and improve their overall quality of life. It's important to work closely with healthcare professionals to develop a personalized care plan and receive ongoing support and guidance throughout the journey.

Chapter 9

Advances in Heart Disease Research

Current Research and Innovations

Researchers continue to explore various aspects of heart disease to improve prevention, diagnosis, and treatment. Some areas of current research include:

Precision Medicine

Advancements in genetics and molecular biology are enabling researchers to better understand the individualized nature of heart disease and develop targeted therapies based on a person's genetic profile.

Biomarkers

Research is focused on identifying and utilizing specific biomarkers that can help in early detection, risk assessment, and monitoring of heart disease. These biomarkers can aid in identifying individuals at high risk and tailoring treatment plans accordingly.

Regenerative Medicine

Scientists are investigating regenerative approaches to repair and replace damaged heart tissue. This includes stem cell therapy, tissue engineering, and other innovative techniques to stimulate heart tissue regeneration and improve heart function.

Artificial Intelligence (AI) and Machine Learning

The use of AI and machine learning algorithms is gaining momentum in heart disease research. These technologies can help analyze vast amounts of data, predict outcomes, and assist in personalized treatment plans.

Emerging Treatments and Therapies

Advancements in research have led to the development of new treatments and therapies for heart disease. Some promising emerging approaches include:

Gene Therapy

Researchers are exploring the use of gene therapy to target and modify specific genes associated with heart disease. This approach aims to correct genetic abnormalities and improve heart function.

Immunotherapy

Immunotherapies, traditionally used in cancer treatment, are being investigated for their potential in managing heart disease. These therapies harness the immune system to target and remove harmful substances or cells involved in heart disease progression.

Nanotechnology

Nanotechnology-based drug delivery systems and devices are being developed to improve the effectiveness and targeted delivery of medications for heart disease. Nanoparticles and nanostructures can enhance drug stability, control release rates, and improve tissue penetration.

Genetic and Molecular Studies

Advances in genetic and molecular studies have shed light on the genetic components and molecular mechanisms underlying heart disease. Researchers are identifying specific genes, genetic variations, and molecular pathways associated with heart disease. This knowledge is essential for understanding disease development, personalizing treatment approaches, and developing targeted therapies.

Genetic Studies

Large-scale genetic studies, such as genome-wide association studies (GWAS), are helping identify genetic variants associated with different types of heart disease. This information aids in risk prediction, early diagnosis, and development of precision medicine approaches.

Molecular Studies

Molecular studies focus on understanding the cellular and molecular processes involved in heart disease. Researchers investigate signaling pathways, protein interactions, and cellular mechanisms to identify potential targets for therapy.

These advances in heart disease research hold the potential to revolutionize the prevention, diagnosis, and treatment of heart disease. However, it's important to note that research findings are still being translated into clinical practice, and further studies are needed to validate their effectiveness and safety. Collaboration between researchers, healthcare professionals, and industry partners is crucial to bringing these innovations to the forefront of patient care.

Conclusion

Heart disease is a prevalent and serious health condition that affects millions of people worldwide. It encompasses various conditions that impact the structure and function of the heart, leading to significant health risks and complications if left untreated. However, with increased awareness and advancements in research and treatment, there is hope for better management and prevention of heart disease.

Key Takeaways

Heart disease encompasses a range of conditions, including coronary artery disease, heart failure, arrhythmias, valvular heart disease, congenital heart disease, cardiomyopathy, and heart infections.

Common risk factors for heart disease include atherosclerosis, hypertension, high cholesterol, diabetes, obesity, smoking, and a family history of heart disease.

Signs and symptoms of heart disease can vary but may include chest pain, shortness of breath, fatigue, palpitations, and swelling in the legs and ankles.

Diagnostic tests and procedures such as electrocardiograms, echocardiograms, stress tests, coronary angiography, and blood tests are used to evaluate heart health and diagnose specific conditions.

Treatment options for heart disease include lifestyle modifications (healthy diet, regular exercise, smoking cessation, stress management), medications, surgical procedures, interventional cardiology, and cardiac rehabilitation.

Prevention and risk reduction strategies include adopting a healthy diet, engaging in regular physical activity, managing blood pressure and cholesterol levels, quitting smoking, controlling diabetes, and practicing stress management.

Importance of Heart Disease Awareness

Raising awareness about heart disease is crucial to educate the public about its risk factors, symptoms, and preventive measures. Awareness campaigns can promote early detection, encourage lifestyle changes, and improve access to healthcare services. By fostering a culture of heart health awareness, individuals can take proactive steps to reduce their risk and seek timely medical attention when needed.

Future Outlook and Heart Health Recommendations

The future of heart disease lies in continued research and innovation. Advances in genetics, molecular studies, regenerative medicine, artificial intelligence, and nanotechnology hold promise for personalized treatments, improved diagnostics, and better outcomes. However, it is essential to prioritize heart health at an individual and societal level. Recommendations for maintaining a healthy heart include:

Adopting and maintaining a heart-healthy lifestyle through nutritious eating, regular physical activity, and stress management.

Engaging in regular health check-ups and monitoring of blood pressure, cholesterol levels, and other relevant parameters.

Seeking support from healthcare professionals, support systems, and resources to manage emotional and psychological aspects of living with heart disease.

Participating in cardiac rehabilitation programs to aid in recovery and improve overall well-being.

Staying informed about advancements in heart disease research and treatment options.

By implementing these recommendations and working

collaboratively with healthcare providers, individuals can take control of their heart health and reduce the burden of heart disease on themselves and society as a whole.

www.ingramcontent.com/pod-product-compliance
Lightning Source LLC
Chambersburg PA
CBHW061514250726
48657CB00005B/1862